Influenza

Epidemics, Pandemics, and Bird Flu

Jane Semple, M.A., N.D.

Dr. J Semple

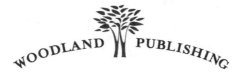

WOODLAND PUBLISHING

For permissions, ordering information, or bulk quantity discounts, please contact: Woodland Publishing, 448 East 800 North, Orem, Utah 84097
Visit our Web site: www.woodlandpublishing.com
Toll-free number: (800) 777-2665

The information in this book is for educational purposes only and is not recommended as a means of diagnosing or treating an illness. All matters concerning physical and mental health should be supervised by a health practitioner knowledgeable in treating that particular condition. Neither the publisher nor the author directly or indirectly dispenses medical advice, nor do they prescribe any remedies or assume any responsibility for those who choose to treat themselves.

ISBN-13: 978-1-58054-425-2
ISBN-10: 1-58054-425-8

Printed in the United States of America

06   07   08   09   10   1   2   3   4   5   6   7   8   9   10

Contents

Viruses and Influenza

A distinction was not made between bacteria and viruses until the early twentieth century. Prior to that time, scientists thought viruses were bacteria small enough to pass through minute pores of a bacteria filter. In addition to their size, the fact that a virus cannot multiply outside of a host cell complicated their detection and identification.

Viruses are parasitic (live off their host) in that they can only reproduce within cells. Viruses enter a cell and take over the cell's machinery, forcing it to manufacture more viruses. Once the virus has exhausted the raw materials in the cell, new viruses are released and attach themselves to new cells. The average time from attachment to release is twenty to forty minutes.

Each new generation allows a virus to mutate or adapt itself to survive in its current environment. Compare twenty to forty minutes to twenty-five to thirty years, the norm for a human generation. A new generation of viruses has an opportunity to mutate or adapt twenty thousand times in a single year.

There are many types of viruses. We will concentrate on influenza, which is second only to the common cold for incidence in developed countries. Symptoms of influenza are chills, fever, headache, and muscle aches. Upper respiratory infection of the lungs and sinuses may also be present. In severe cases there may be a cough. Diarrhea is not a typical symptom of the flu. Intestinal discomfort attributed to the "stomach flu" is probably from some other cause, like bacteria in food or "food poisoning." A runny nose is more characteristic of the common cold.

Three Types of Influenza Virus

According to the Centers for Disease Control and Prevention (CDC), there are three types of influenza viruses: A, B, and C. A-type viruses are responsible for major pandemics (epidemics that occur worldwide). B-type viruses also circulate and mutate, but usually cause milder infections. C-type viruses cause mild illness in humans.

The influenza virus consists of eight links of RNA segments enclosed in an inner layer of protein and an outer layer of lipid (fat). Embedded in the lipid layer are projections, hemagglutinin (H), and neuraminidase (N) spikes. The H spikes allow the virus to recognize and attach to the body. The N spikes help the virus separate from the infected cell after reproduction. Antibodies produced by our immune system against the influenza virus are mainly directed at these spikes. Pharmaceutical drugs and herbs are also believed to work by inactivating the H or N spikes.

Viruses are classified into strains using the H and N spikes as identifiers. An Influenza A virus identified as H1N1 was isolated in 1933, H2N2 in the Asiatic pandemic of 1957, H3N2 in the Hong Kong pandemic of 1968, and H1N1 for the swine flu of 1976. According to the CDC, the strains circulating in 2006 include H1N1, H1N2, and H3N2. According to the World Health Organization (WHO), a strain identified as H5N1 has jumped from host species (birds) to humans, though it does not appear to be easily passed from human to human as of May 2006. Influenza Type-B and Influenza Type-C are not classified according to subtype.

Viruses are further classified as having low pathogenic potential or high pathogenic potential. Low pathogenic strains are associated with mild disease, while high pathogenic strains can cause severe illness and may have a high mortality rate. There is always potential for low pathogenic forms to mutate into high pathogenic forms. The eight RNA segments of a virus can recombine, creating new strains.

Drifts are small, gradual changes, while shifts are abrupt, major changes. A person or animal may become infected with more than one strain, encouraging recombination and genetic shifts. A person or animal with multiple strains is called a "mixing vessel" that is responsible for new strains.

The result of a shift is that antibodies produced by the body for older strains may not confer immunity for newer strains. In addition, a vaccine or drug effective against one strain will be less effective or completely ineffective against a new mutation.

"Bird Flu" and Influenza Pandemics

Most viruses are able to infect only one species (birds, pigs, horses, seals, or humans). We hear a lot of hype about the "bird flu" or "avian flu." Wild birds (avians) are the natural hosts for all Influenza Type-A viruses, so most pandemics are "bird flu." Wild birds do not typically become ill, but can pass illness on to domestic poultry, especially through their feces.

Domestic poultry such as turkeys and chickens can become infected from water or feed that have been contaminated with strains of a wild bird virus. Influenza A can cross over from domestic birds to other species, usually pigs or humans. Transmission to a human can occur among persons who are in direct contact with infected birds, especially feces, blood, or mucus. Another route is transmission to pigs and then to humans. Pigs are a frequent intermediate host, thus the term "swine flu," though the initial carrier was a bird. Additional mutations are usually required for the strain to be spread through human-to-human contact.

Influenza Pandemic of 1918

An influenza pandemic started in 1918 and continued into 1919. Some historians believe that it started at Fort Riley, Kansas, and was spread throughout Europe by U.S. servicemen. Others believe the pandemic started in European military camps, spread by soldiers returning home.

While the origins of this pandemic were debated, one inescapable fact is that it was deadly. According to Michael Osterholm, M.P.H., Ph.D., a world-renowned infectious disease specialist, the 1918 pandemic killed over one hundred million people worldwide, including about one million Americans. Even in years with less virulent strains, flu kills thirty-six thousand people every year in the United States alone.

The H/N classification system had not yet been devised in 1918. However, through a miracle of modern technology, Dr. Osterholm explains that the Armed Forces Institute of Pathology was able to recreate the 1918 virus. Tissue was recovered from old slides of patients who had died and whose bodies were exhumed in an Alaskan village. With the material collected, Jeffery Taubenberger and his group were able to reassemble the eight genes of the 1918 virus. The 2006 H5N1 influenza virus is considered a close cousin to the 1918 strain.

New Strains of Influenza, Epidemics, and Pandemics

In recent years, new flu strains have been originating in Asia with some regularity. Authorities believe the close proximity of birds, pigs, and people contributes to antigenic shifts (major, abrupt changes). Pigs make especially good mixing vessels, combining bird and human viruses into new, virulent strains.

Newly mutated strains of the flu that spread rapidly through large, local populations are referred to as an epidemic. They become a pandemic as they spread throughout the world due to the pervasiveness of air travel. Public health officials report that the increase in global travel is making influenza outbreaks more common. The speed and frequency of modern travel makes controlling pandemics more difficult.

Though deadly strains can occur, symptoms of the flu are usually mild, lasting only a few days, with mortality less than 1 percent. The very young, very old, and those with heart or lung ailments or compromised immune systems are most susceptible. The pandemic of 1918 was different in that mortality was high among twenty- to forty-year-olds. The fact that the flu spread among servicemen in cramped military camps is a possible cause for the high mortality among young men.

Dr. Osterholm estimates that a pandemic with a highly pathogenic influenza strain, similar to 1918, would kill 180 million to 360 million people worldwide. In the United States, he believes 90 million people would become ill, and 2 million would die. Pandemics do not last for just a few weeks; they come in waves for a year or two.

Antibiotics and Influenza—A Losing Battle

Influenza infections are usually restricted to the upper respiratory system, but may invade the lungs causing viral pneumonia. Antibiotics are not indicated and will not help viral pneumonia. Antibiotics must be used with discretion and only when appropriate. Overuse of antibiotics is causing bacteria to mutate, which is creating antibacterial-resistant bacteria. Resistant bacteria become more virulent, endangering future generations.

> Every time you take an antibiotic,
> you are killing one of your grandchildren!

I made this comment to a pharmaceutical professor in a conventional medical class I was taking. He said he agreed with the premise, though he did not think it would take that long. In other words, you are endangering your children as well. I made the same comment to a pathophysiology (study of disease) professor, and she said, "Wow, that's pretty profound," agreeing wholeheartedly.

Pharmaceutical Drugs

According to the most recent *Physician's Drug Handbook*, the following are approved to treat influenza.

Antivirals

Amantadine/Symmetrel is classified as an antiviral, but is also used for Parkinson's disease. Amantadine is believed to interfere with viral uncoating. Adverse reactions include anxiety, confusion, depression, dizziness, fatigue, hallucinations, headache, insomnia, irritability, light-headedness, heart failure, hypotension, constipation, dry mouth, nausea, and vomiting. Amantadine also interacts with alcohol and stimulants.

Rimantadine/Flumadine is classified as an antiviral approved for use in various strains of Influenza A. This drug is believed to inhibit viral replication by interfering with viral uncoating. Rimantadine must be started within forty-eight hours of onset. Adverse reactions include dizziness, fatigue, headache, impaired concentration, insomnia, nervousness, abdominal pain, dry mouth, nausea, and vomiting. Spontaneous resistance is common, and the drug loses its effectiveness against an Influenza A strain.

Oseltamivir/Tamiflu is an antiviral that is believed to inhibit an enzyme of Influenza A and B used in replication and inhibit viral release from the host. Adverse reactions include dizziness, fatigue, headache, insomnia, vertigo, abdominal pain, diarrhea, nausea, vomiting, bronchitis, and cough.

Zanamivir/Relenza is an antiviral that acts much like Tamiflu, inhibiting an enzyme used in replication and inhibiting viral release from the host cell. Adverse reactions include dizziness, headache, ear infections, sore throat, sinusitis, diarrhea, nausea, vomiting, bronchitis, and cough.

The side effects of these medications sound strangely like the flu! Even minor mutations, antigenic drifts, mean available vaccines introduced later and pharmaceutical drugs will no longer be effective.

In January 2006, the Centers for Disease Control and Prevention (CDC) issued a warning urging doctors not to prescribe amantadine and rimantadine due to resistance of the current strains of Influenza A. "Clinicians should not use rimantadine and amantadine because the drugs will not be effective," said CDC Director Dr. Julie Gerberding. Of the 2006 strains, 91 percent were resistant to the two drugs. In 2004 only 2 percent were resistant, while 11 percent of the strains were resistant in 2005.

It appears that oseltamivir/Tamiflu and zanamivir/Relenza are at least somewhat effective against the late 2005 strain. However, Dr. Osterholm reports that they are not nearly as effective against the 2006 bird flu mutation in Turkey. In addition, they need to be started within hours of onset or the drugs will not be effective. Use of pharmaceutical drugs for low-pathogenic strains actually encourage resistant mutations, so it might be best to wait and use these antiviral drugs for the "big one."

Vaccines

An influenza virus vaccine is available by injection and as a mist. This vaccine is changed yearly to include viruses prevalent at the time of manufacture. Adverse reactions include fever, headache, irritability, tiredness, weakness, nasal congestion, ear infection, sinusitis, sore throat, abdominal pain, diarrhea, vomiting, muscle aches, cough, and chills.

People have varying degrees of success with vaccines. I do not generally recommend them for my clients, though each person should make their own decision. I would never take one myself, even for a highly pathogenic strain.

Dr. Osterholm states, "We're not going to have a vaccine. Modern medicine is not going to save us." A vaccine must be designed with the current strain. In an entire year, worldwide capability of vaccine production is about three hundred million, or 5 percent of the world population.

I had an older part-time employee who resisted getting a flu shot and never missed a day of work. One year she let her physician talk her into being immunized and was out sick for three weeks. She said she could not imagine being sicker if she had gotten the flu itself.

Another client let her physician talk her and her husband into getting flu shots, presumably because the husband had a heart condition and might not survive a bad bout of flu. Both became so ill from the immunization that I had to treat them for the flu. It took a week for the wife to recover and nearly two weeks for her husband to recover. I assume it took longer for the husband to recover because he wasted a week taking a prescription drug before switching to herbs.

A local physician started using the FluMist vaccine in 2004, as an alternative to injections. Her patients certainly appreciated the easy administration of a spray. The problem is that the mist is a live agent, and was being administered in the office. So, they ended up with live flu virus throughout their exam rooms, offices, and waiting room. The entire staff and anyone visiting their office got the flu. Every surface had to be disinfected.

Influenza Has Been a Formidable Opponent to Conventional Medicine

These are clear examples of why conventional medicine does not work. Drugs are too simplistic, readily allowing pathogens to mutate, developing immunity. Immunizations may or may not work, sometimes causing flu symptoms.

During the 1918 influenza pandemic, posters instructing citizens on precautions they should take were plastered throughout the nation. Recommendations included: chew foods carefully and avoid tight clothes and shoes. There were also many helpful suggestions like avoiding the use of common utensils, frequent washing of hands, and attention to general hygiene. People were cautioned against exhaustion and encouraged to get fresh air. (PBS)

There Are Alternative Solutions

I have the utmost respect for emergency medicine in the United States and Canada. Accident victims are truly fortunate to have well-trained medical professionals available. However, conventional medicine fails miserably when it comes to common illnesses. Pharmaceutical drugs may do more harm than good, working only for a year or two before encouraging more virulent strains as the viruses develop resistance.

Medicines and herbs from nature are too complicated for pathogens to "find their way around." In the 1918 pandemic, there were reports of people warding off the flu or recovering from the flu with onions and garlic, though I do not recommend that you rely on these alone.

This failure of conventional medicine has led people worldwide to seek alternatives to protect themselves against contracting the flu. Many herbs with proven safety records can improve immune function, protect against the flu, diminish symptoms, and reduce the length and severity of the flu. Although this book focuses on the flu, most recommendations are appropriate for the common cold as well.

There is no guarantee that any one individual will be saved through alternative means. This book is about giving you a fighting chance. If there is a pandemic, I will be working through it (assuming I am not sick). I will not be hiding out in my home.

Major Herbs

Astragalus (*Astragalus membranaceus*) is important in Traditional Chinese Medicine as an immune booster and adaptogen. It is known as *Huang Chi* or "yellow energy." Its numerous potential therapeutic applications are beyond the scope of this book, but astragalus has been successfully used to fight viruses that cause colds and flu.

Because viruses depend on their host cells for replication, it is difficult to inhibit viral replication without damaging the host cell itself. One way the body inhibits viral replication is with interferons. Interferons are a class of antiviral proteins produced by cells after viral stimulation. Astragalus has been shown to enhance interferon production, as well as stimulating T-cells and natural killer cells.

Bacteria are often opportunistic infections that are able to reproduce when one's immune system is compromised. Astragalus, as well as many herbs profiled here, has demonstrated antibacterial activity. Herbs and immune-boosting nutrients may help reduce secondary bacterial infections associated with the flu.

Echinacea is a member of the sunflower family, with nine species found in the United States and Canada. Three of the most common species have a long history of medicinal use: *Echinacea angustifolia* (narrow-leafed purple coneflower), *Echinacea pallida* (pale purple coneflower), and *Echinacea purpurea* (purple coneflower).

There are hundreds of research studies on the medicinal uses of echinacea. Two of its major uses are to boost the immune system and inhibit viruses. This herb is used to reduce the length and severity of cold and flu symptoms. Echinacea root or plant may be powdered and put into capsules or pressed into tablets. Echinacea may also be preserved as a glycerin or alcohol extract.

The outcomes of clinical trials on echinacea have been mixed. This is likely due to the use of various species, part of the plant used, preparation, dosage, and how quickly treatment was started. Most studies report a positive outcome.

A few studies have compared a high-dose and low-dose of echinacea against a placebo for cold and flu viruses. Only the high-dose group had a reduction in length and severity of symptoms compared to the placebo group. A few studies started treatment only after a doctor verified the illness. Verification took up to three days from illness onset. It is important that treatment is started within the first four hours of onset of illness and that the dosage be sufficient.

The World Health Organization (WHO) recommends 3,000 mg of *Echinacea angustifolia* daily, yet a study in the November 2005 issue of the *New England Journal of Medicine* used a dose of only 900 mg daily. The researchers further produced their own extract rather than using a commercially available brand. If you want to design research to show that something doesn't work, there are ways of doing so, such as using the wrong part of the plant, using too small a dose, or starting treatment too late. The negative publicity of the 2005 study did not reduce my sales of echinacea products. Those who use this herb know it works.

The German Commission E and the World Health Organization approve *Echinacea purpurea* and *Echinacea pallida* for use in colds and influenza-like infections. These two species are also recommended to strengthen resistance to infections especially in the upper respiratory tract.

As effective as echinacea is, it is not a miracle cure, and I find it works better in combination with other herbs. If you are using echinacea alone, consider doubling or tripling the bottle's dosage recommendation for the first day or two, then reducing it to the recommended dosage. Large oral doses are considered safe.

If you find that echinacea doesn't work for you, be sure you are using a good brand. Some herbs are cut with fillers like rice powder. Raw materials that are refused by larger companies due to poor quality are simply sold to other companies. Also consider using echinacea as I suggest, in combination with other herbs.

Echinacea is not recommended for people with autoimmune diseases, due to its immune stimulating effect. I have suggested combinations with this herb for short-term use in colds and flu, as well as patients with multiple sclerosis and rheumatoid arthritis with no exacerbation of symptoms. If you have been diagnosed with an autoimmune disease, use echinacea carefully.

The **Elder** (*Sambucus nigra*) is a small tree related to the honeysuckle, native to Europe, Asia, and North Africa, which has been naturalized in the United States and Canada. The flower and berry are the parts used.

Elder flowers and elderberries may be powdered and put into capsules or pressed into chewable tablets that have a sweet/tart taste acceptable to children.

Elder is used for colds and flu. The German Commission E approves its use for fevers and to increase bronchial secretions in respiratory infections. Research shows that the mechanism of action of elder is in inhibiting the H spikes, which a virus uses to attach itself to cells.

Garlic (*Allium sativum*) contains a compound called allicin, one of the plant kingdom's most potent, broad-spectrum antibiotics. Its aromatic compounds are readily released into the lungs and respiratory tract. Garlic is one of the few herbs that has achieved universal usage and recognition. It may be used as a preventative for most infectious disease or during illness to fight pathogenic organisms.

Garlic can be used cooked or raw, powdered, prepared as an oil or tincture, or the cloves can just be eaten. If you have friends and wish to keep them, I don't recommend overusing garlic. As wonderful as it is, it also teams up well with just about any other herb to fight the flu.

Garlic can be used for babies and young children by rubbing a little on the bottom of their feet. Mix the garlic with a little olive oil to prevent irritation. For a small baby, if the soles of the feet get red, wipe off the excess garlic with a cloth, and then apply more olive oil to reduce the concentration.

Goldenseal (*Hydrastis canadensis*) is a member of the buttercup family, found in the wild in the eastern and northwest United States. Wild sources are diminishing for this important therapeutic herb so home cultivation is encouraged.

A component of goldenseal, berberine, appears to assist white blood cells in destroying viruses and bacteria. It can be used singly, but is usually used in combination with echinacea. Goldenseal is generally encapsulated in powdered form or prepared as a tincture. Goldenseal should be used carefully, and for less than seven to ten days.

Goldenseal may reduce blood sugar levels. If you are diabetic with hypoglycemic (low sugar) episodes, use goldenseal with caution. Goldenseal is not for long-term use, in any case.

Olive Leaf (*Olea europa*) has a long history of use in Mediterranean cultures, being used in ancient Egypt for nutritional and medicinal purposes. Olive leaves were historically used to treat fevers and malaria.

Upjohn stirred widespread interest in researching olive leaf extract in the 1960s. This extract has shown remarkable antiviral action against colds, flu, and other viral infections. In fact, olive leaf was successful in inhibiting the growth of every virus it was tested against.

Teas are not considered to be as effective as guaranteed-potency capsules or tablets, which are usually 5 to 23 percent oleuropein per dose. Oleuropein is a major antiviral alkaloid (component). Another component, elenolic acid, has also demonstrated impressive antiviral properties.

Minor Herbs

Do not let the term "minor" mislead you. The following herbs are important in treating influenza, but usually play a supporting role.

Catnip (*Nepeta cataria*) is a traditional cold, flu, and bronchitis remedy. It is a diaphoretic (promotes sweating) used in feverish conditions. It is an excellent remedy for children. Usually used in combinations.

Cayenne (*Capsicum annuum*) increases circulation. This herb is often used in combinations to increase the action of the other herbs and get them into the system more quickly. It has a history of use as a gargle for sore throats and laryngitis. I have several clients who swear by this remedy for throat conditions. They add a little capsicum tincture to water and use it as a gargle or squirt a little capsicum on their throat then take a few sips of water.

Chickweed (*Stellaria media*) is a cousin to the carnation, found in the wild from the equator to the Arctic Circle. It is considered a garden pest, but has many medicinal uses.

Colloidal Silver is an excellent antimicrobial, inhibiting viruses, bacteria, fungi, and protozoa. Reports claim it inhibits 650 pathogens. Colloidal silver is reported to work without side effects and without damaging the cells of the body. It is virtually tasteless, so you don't have to fight with your children to get them to take it.

Silver can be taken orally or atomized and inhaled. I recommend using it only as needed for seven to ten days at a time, not continuously. I sometimes suggest using colloidal silver as part of a supplement program when an illness does not respond to an herbal combination or when someone has waited until they are "really" sick before coming in.

Eleuthero (*Eleutherococcus senticosus*) was formerly called Siberian ginseng. Two Russian studies suggest it can greatly reduce the incidence of influenza and colds. A study of thirteen thousand auto plant employees showed that eleuthero reduced infections by 40 percent. Another study of one thousand mining employees reduced acute respiratory diseases by nearly half. (Beckman, 1980)

Ephedra (*Ephedra sinica*) is an evergreen shrub native to central Asia. In Asian medicine, ephedra is a major herb used in the treatment of asthma and bronchitis.

There has been considerable controversy about this herb in the United States, mainly due to individuals abusing ephedra as a diet aid and to enhance athletic performance. Ephedra is considered safe when used in small doses for brief periods of time. It should not be mixed with other stimulants including caffeine and caffeine-like substances such as guaraná, kola nut, sodas, coffee, and excessive tea. You should be under the care of a qualified alternative health-care professional for high-dose or long-term use of this herb.

Alkaloids (chemical components) of ephedra have been synthesized by the pharmaceutical industry and used as drugs, including ephedrine and pseudoephedrine. These alkaloids are used in over-the-counter diet aids and cold medications. The entire herb is better tolerated than its synthetic components.

I have recommended ephedra in small doses for occasional use for asthma and sinus congestion. One elderly client was taking a small dose two to three times daily for chronic obstructive pulmonary disease, a degenerative disease of the lungs. After a point, the small dose was no longer sufficient, so I increased her dosage to a 20 mg capsule.

This dose is high enough to be used as a diet aid. She stayed on that dosage for five years, with no ill effects. She was not on a single pharmaceutical drug at that time. When she went into a nursing home, they took away her ephedra "because it was dangerous." She died about a year later—on multiple drugs to try to control her lung disease.

Fenugreek (*Trigonella foenum-graecum*) soothes inflamed tissues. It softens and dissolves thickened mucus to clear lungs and sinuses. Fenugreek has a long history of use in respiratory infections including influenza, colds, and asthma. This herb also promotes sweating, lowering fever and helping toxins move through the skin, which reduces strain on the other excretory organs.

Ginger (*Zingiber officinale*) contains nearly a dozen antiviral compounds. Ginger also contains alkaloids, chemical components that reduce pain and fever, settle the stomach, and suppress cough.

Ginger may be encapsulated or taken as a tea. Ginger ale has long been used for nausea. I remember my mother, a registered nurse, saying that ginger ale seemed to work, while 7-Up did not. This is likely due to the fact that ginger settles the stomach. I recommend my clients purchase a name-brand product. I recall an old commercial, "Real Ginger from Jamaica." A good brand of ginger ale will likely contain ginger, not an artificial flavor substitute.

Horseradish (*Armoracia rusticana*) is in the mustard family. It is a home remedy used for influenza and fevers. A dose of horseradish will clear the sinuses. It can be powdered and encapsulated, or the chopped root can be infused as a tea or spread on a sandwich. Horseradish is a stimulant similar to cayenne and is often used in combinations.

Lobelia (*Lobelia inflata*) is a respiratory stimulant, primarily used in bronchitis and bronchial asthma. Lobelia relaxes the muscles of the respiratory system and should be considered whenever breathing is a problem.

Powdered lobelia may be encapsulated and taken alone or in herbal combinations. A liquid extract may be taken sublingually (under the tongue) when quick action is needed. For small children, consider rubbing a liquid extract of lobelia on the soles of the feet. If a liquid extract is not available, a capsule can be opened and mixed with olive oil, then rubbed on the soles of the feet.

Excess lobelia may cause nausea, so it's best used in small, repeated doses until the desired effect is achieved. The overall action is actually a combination of stimulation and relaxation.

Marshmallow (*Althaea officinalis*) has been used as a soothing herb for sore throats and respiratory conditions and is endorsed by the German Commission E. Okra is in the same family. For throats, marshmallow is best used as a tea or lozenge. The leaf is usually used for ailments of the lungs and urinary system, though the leaves have similar qualities to the root.

The puffy white treats we are familiar with were named "marshmallow" after this herb. The marshmallow herb contains spongy mucilage that soothes soft tissue, thus the name for the soft, spongy treat. For sore throat that may accompany the flu, use the herb marshmallow, though the sugary marshmallows do go well in hot cocoa.

Meadowsweet (*Spiraea ulmaria*) is also called queen of the meadow. This fragrant perennial herb is native to Europe and Asia, but has been naturalized in the United States and Canada.

Salicylic acid, or aspirin, was first synthesized from meadowsweet. Aspirin owes its name to this herb's Latin genus, *Spiraea*. Meadowsweet should be avoided in severe aspirin allergies.

Commission E has approved its use as a supportive therapy for colds or feverish conditions. This is not a major flu herb, but may be found as a minor herb in combinations. It is one of the many herbs indicated in fever.

Mullein (*Verbascum thapsus*) is soothing to the throat and is also used as an expectorant. This plant may have antiviral properties that inhibit flu. Mullein is useful for any respiratory ailment, as it is soothing to swollen membranes. Flowers or leaves may be powdered in a capsule or used as a tea. An extract made with olive oil is useful for earaches.

Mushrooms, including reishi, maitake, and cordyceps, have antioxidant and immune-stimulating properties. I usually stay with recommending herbs for influenza, but occasionally suggest a combination that contains one or more mushrooms.

Myrrh (*Commiphora molmol*) is a bush indigenous to Asia and East Africa. The myrrh bush secretes a resin that is collected and used medicinally. Myrrh aids the immune system and has both antiviral and antibacterial properties.

The resin may be powdered and encapsulated or taken as a tea, though it is an acquired taste. Myrrh is used much like goldenseal, and may be substituted for goldenseal in combinations for those with hypoglycemia (low blood sugar) or diabetics with hypoglycemic episodes.

Onion (*Allium cepa*) is a cousin of garlic, containing many similar antiviral compounds. The humble onion is a native of Asia, but is now grown throughout the world. Onions can be eaten cooked or raw. The white onion is the strongest and most pungent, the yellow is milder, while the red and purple are the mildest. Consider steeping raw onions in honey overnight then put a tablespoon of the mixture in a cup of herbal tea to soothe an irritated throat and reduce cough.

Pleurisy Root (*Asclepias tuberosa*), as its name implies, is effective against respiratory infections. It is used to treat influenza, bronchitis, and pleurisy, assisting in expectoration. It combines well with cayenne and lobelia.

Royal Jelly is synthesized by worker bees exclusively for the nourishment of the queen. Even though she is hatched from the same egg as a honeybee, she will live four to five years, compared to one or two months for the honeybee.

Royal jelly and another bee product, propolis, have many therapeutic actions, including stimulating the immune system. Royal jelly, propolis, and to some extent bee pollen and honey, are considered to have antiviral and antibacterial properties. Bee products combine well with eleuthero and ginseng.

There is always a potential for an allergic reaction to any bee product, so use caution if you are allergic to bee stings.

Slippery Elm Bark (*Ulmus fulva*) is even approved by the FDA as a safe and effective treatment for sore throats and respiratory ailments. This herb can also be used to suppress cough and soothe the intestines. It can be powdered and put into capsules for respiratory and intestinal distress, but it is best pressed into lozenges or used as a tea for throat ailments.

Thyme (*Thymus vulgaris*) is a small shrub with small lavender flowers. Thyme has antiseptic properties primarily due to the volatile oils it contains. This common cooking herb is used to treat respiratory ailments, as it dilates the bronchioles. Thyme is also used for sore or scratchy throats and coughs.

Willow Bark (*Salix alba* or *Salix purpurea*) is a shrub native to Asia, Europe, and North America. It is used to reduce fevers and relieve pain, much as meadowsweet. Avoid this herb in severe aspirin allergies.

Yarrow (*Achillea millefolium*) is native to Europe but has taken well to North America, and is seen nearly everywhere as a weed or as a popular perennial in flower beds. Yarrow is a standard remedy for fevers, because it promotes sweating. Yarrow is said to keep wounds from becoming inflamed.

As with other herbs, chemical content varies with the part of the plant, its age, season, and environmental conditions, so you may not get the results you want from an ornamental species. There have been some rare allergic reactions, perhaps because yarrow contains a small amount of salicylic acid, from which aspirin is derived. This herb combines well with elderberry, elder flower, cayenne, and ginger.

Vitamins and Minerals

Vitamin C, also known as ascorbic acid, has been clinically proven to reduce the length and severity of colds and flu. The amount individuals can absorb through the intestinal tract varies, so be careful not to take dosages beyond your bowel's tolerance or it can cause diarrhea.

I was taking a "nutrition" class at a local college, which was part of the required program for nurses and a few other medical specialties. I was appalled when our textbook reported a study where vitamin C only reduced the length of a cold by a few hours, so it was hardly worth taking. I looked up the study and found they were giving participants either 100 mg of vitamin C or a placebo. This is not a typo—it was only 100 mg. Our instructor agreed that 100 mg is the maximum a body can absorb, and any more would just cause diarrhea.

During our next class, I brought in a bottle of 1,000 mg time-released vitamin C. At the beginning of a three-hour class I took three 1,000 mg tablets. At the end of the class the instructor was surprised that I was not experiencing any intestinal irritation.

For a cold or flu, consider taking 1,000 mg of vitamin C two to six times daily, depending upon your history with this vitamin. There is no reason to cause discomfort. Be sure you are also taking herbs, as there is no one magic bullet for the treatment of influenza.

Zinc promotes a healthy immune system and is a constituent of many important enzymes, including superoxide dismutase (SOD). Zinc has been reported to be effective in reducing the length and severity of colds and flu.

Don't forget other immune building vitamins and minerals. Be sure to get sufficient amounts of vitamins A and E, B-complex, carotenes, and oligameric proanthocyanidin complexes (OPCs) derived from grape seeds and pine bark (Pycnogenol), as well as the antioxidant mineral selenium.

Greens

Green drinks are a great way to boost immune function. You may take greens as a preventative or during illness. Some greens are now encapsulated, for those of us who prefer them that way. Many good green products are available, including some of the following:

Amaranth contains antioxidants, folic acid, carotenes, calcium and trace minerals; seeds are high in protein, lignans, and protease inhibitors.

Barley grass is rich in chlorophyll, lignans, and protease inhibitors.

Lemongrass is rich in chlorophyll, lignans, and protease inhibitors.

Spirulina is high in protein, the essential fatty acid GLA, vitamin B-12 (not usually available in non-animal sources) and is high in chlorophyll.

Wheatgrass has a nutritional value that is claimed to be twenty-five times greater than the choicest vegetables and is high in chlorophyll.

Chlorophyll taken as a liquid can also be quite helpful. Just squirt a few drops in warm or cold water for a minty taste.

Juices

Several concentrated fruit juices are available, such as:

Noni (*Morinda citrifolia*)

Mangosteen (*Garcinia mangostana*)

Goji, or Wolfberry (*Lycium barbarum*)

These juices are from exotic places and are not readily available as whole fruits. All have high amounts of antioxidants, which have antiviral properties.

Adult dosage is usually one ounce straight or in water, once or twice per day. I usually recommend a tablespoon for young children, more for those twelve or older.

Essential Oils

In addition to herbs and nutritional supplements, essential oils can be important in treating influenza. We use essential oils in our office to reduce the spread of pathogens. We spray a combination into the air through an atomizer, and add oils to liquid hand soap and cleaning solutions.

Essential oils are applied topically (on the skin), atomized into the air, or added to cleaning solutions. *Do not* drink essential oils, as large quantities can be dangerous. They are, however, considered safe when used as suggested. For babies and small children please consult a natural health practitioner familiar with the use of oils.

Try one essential oil at a time if you have a lot of allergies and sensitivities. One client did have a reaction to eucalyptus. It was the only problem I have had, and I no longer use eucalyptus in our atomizer. Clients comment on the clean smell in our office and love our liquid hand soap.

Basil is spicy and refreshing; used for bronchitis, fatigue, colds, aches, and pains.

Bergamot has a fresh, fruity scent used for coughs, colds, and fevers.

Eucalyptus has a fresh, penetrating scent; often component of liniments, salves, and cold-care products; used for sore throats, coughs, and sinusitis and as an antiseptic; careful of allergic reactions, they are rare but possible.

Frankincense has a sweet, balsamic aroma used extensively in incense and fine perfumery; used for sores, wounds, and as an antiseptic.

Lavender, with a sweet, floral fragrance, can be used directly on the skin; used for headaches, insomnia and tension; considered safe for babies and small children.

Lemon has a fresh, fruity scent; a great addition to household antiseptic products; also used for sore throats; considered safe for babies and small children.

Oregano has a warm, herbaceous scent; used for viral and respiratory infections; excellent antifungal.

Spearmint has a potent, fresh, minty fragrance; used as a digestive tonic in nausea, body aches, and headaches.

Tea Tree has a spicy, penetrating scent; excellent for viral, bacterial, and fungal infections.

Thyme has a spicy, herbaceous scent; used for viral and bacterial infections and to improve immune function.

Essential Oil Combinations: Any of the following combinations can be mixed with 1 tablespoon of carrier oil and applied to the chest. For a young child, consider applying to the bottom of the feet. You may add essential oils to a hot bath, with or without carrier oil. Carrier oils include apricot kernel, grape seed, sweet almond, and olive oil. If applied oil is irritating to the skin, dilute with more carrier oil, *not* water. Oil and water do not mix, so water will not dilute oil.

Choose one of the following formulas or make up your own:

- 2 drops thyme, 2 tea tree or oregano,
    2 eucalyptus or bergamot, 2 lemon
- 2 drops oregano, 2 bergamot or eucalyptus,
    2 frankincense, 2 lemon
- 3 drops oregano, 1 thyme or basil,
    2 peppermint or spearmint

Essential oils can be atomized directly into the air. Do not dilute with carrier oil, as this will leave a sticky residue. Lemon or lavender provide a good base. Use 1/2 to 3/4 parts lemon or lavender then add any two additional oils depending upon your preference. Mix a small amount of oil initially, so you do not end up with something you consider "stinky."

Cleaning with Essential Oils: Start with a natural, dye-free base. Hand Soap: 1/4 base, 3/4 water to equal 16 ounces. In hand soap dispenser: 10 drops lemon, peppermint, or spearmint; 10 drops bergamot or lavender. Use a combination of at least three oils. Do not use the same combination continuously. You may also add essential oils directly to any commercial soap product.

For cleaning counter surfaces use hand soap, then add a few drops of basil, frankincense, oregano, tea tree, or thyme. For floors, add a few extra drops.

What You Can Do to Prepare for the Flu

Be prepared instead of panicking in the middle of a pandemic. Have a stock of herbs and vitamins at home. It is important that you begin treatment at the first sign of the flu. If you feel ill during the night, you cannot wait until the stores open in the morning. Remember, the virus is multiplying every twenty to forty minutes. The quicker you get started, the better chance you have of getting well.

Purchase a few extra herbs and vitamins that you can use in the meantime for any cold or flu. Just be sure you keep up your stock. When the "big" bird flu hits North America, your local health food store may have difficulty keeping sufficient stock of flu remedies on the shelves. I have run out of some popular flu products temporarily even during a "typical" flu season.

If you do not feel qualified to treat yourself, find a local naturopath or herbalist *now* and develop a relationship. Do not wait until you have something contagious before you schedule an appointment. Have an initial consultation, for which you should expect to pay a fee. You should not expect to speak to someone over the telephone for a list of recommendations, except on a fee basis. Ask for credentials, you want someone with both training and experience.

Many health food stores have knowledgeable employees. States vary on how permissive they are regarding the fine line between recommending and practicing medicine without a license. Store employees will be more open with you once they get to know you. So, find a store you like and become a regular customer.

At my office, new clients must schedule an appointment so I can collect a history and build a file on them. My office manager keeps track of all product purchases, so we know by looking at their file what products they have at home. I do not under any circumstance make recommendations over the telephone except for regular clients.

I, for one, will not go to an emergency room. I consider hospitals a good place to pick up resistant viruses and bacteria. I have not taken a pharmaceutical drug for over seventeen years and would not take one for the flu, as I have complete confidence in herbs and my own abilities.

I am not promising everyone a cure, just a fighting chance.

How to Locate a Practitioner

For a natural health-care practitioner near you, check your local phone directory under Naturopaths, Herbs, or Alternative Medicine. Naturopaths, herbalists, and health food store employees will be familiar with standard flu remedies. You may also contact the American Naturopathic Medical Association (ANMA), PO Box 96273, Las Vegas, NV, 89193, 702-897-7053. The ANMA is the oldest and largest naturopathic association, with approximately four thousand members.

Bibliography

Barney, Paul, M.D. *Doctor's Guide to Natural Medicine*. Orem, UT: Woodland Publishing, 1998.

"Bird Flu: The Untold Story." Transcript from the *Oprah Winfrey Show*, Chicago: Harpo Productions, January 24, 2006.

Blumenthal, Mark, Alicia Goldberg, and Josef Brinckmann. *Herbal Medicine: Expanded Commission E Monographs*. Austin: American Botanical Council, 2000.

Brekhman, H. "Eleutherococcus: 20 Years of Research and Clinical Application."Presentation at the First International Symposium on Eleutherococcus, Hamburg, Germany, May, 1980.

Duke, James, Ph.D. *Green Pharmacy*. Emmaus, PA: Rodale Press, 1997.

Elkins, Rita, M.H. *Healing From the Hive*. Orem, UT: Woodland Publishing, 1996.

Fillon, Mike. *Ephedra Fact & Fiction*. Orem, UT: Woodland Publishing, 2003.

German Federal Institute for Drugs and Medical Devices Commission E, American Botanical Council, et al. *Complete German Commission E Monograph*. Austin: American Botanical Council, 1998.

Herb Allure Resource Toolkit. Jamestown, NY: Herb Allure, 2004.

Herbalgram: The Journal of the American Botanical Council, January 2006.

Hoffman, David. *New Holistic Herbal*. Boston: Element Books, 1990.

Kowalchik, Claire and William H. Hylton, eds. *Rodale's Illustrated Encyclopedia of Herbs*. Emmaus, PA: Rodale Press, 1987.

Ritchason, Jack, N.D. *Olive Leaf Extract*. Orem, UT: Woodland Publishing, 1999.

Satterlee, David. *Health Education Library*. League City, TX.

Tortora, Gerard J., Christine L. Case, and Berdell L. Funke. *Microbiology*, Sixth Edition. Menlo Park, CA: Benjamin Cummings Publishing, 1988.

Twenty Essential Supplements for Super Health. Orem, UT: Woodland Publishing, 2005.

Worwood, Valerie Ann. *Complete Book of Essential Oils and Aromatherapy*. Novato, CA: New World Library, 1991.

Web Sites

American Botanical Council: www.herbalgram.org

PBS American Experience : www.pbs.org/wghb/amex/influenza

U.S. Government Centers for Disease Control and Prevention: www.cdc.gov; www.cdc.gov/flu/avian/index.htm ; www.pamdemicflu.gov

World Health Organization: www.who.int/csr/disease